THE MINISTRY OF CAREGIVING

Are you a believer caring for a sick loved one? Be encouraged! Care-giving is a ministry calling. You have been called, chosen and commissioned by God to provide healthcare for your sick loved one. Yes, care-giving is a ministry and God is able to supply you with the spiritual, practical and emotional skills needed to perform this task in love.

SPIRITUALLY

As humans, we are three-fold beings. We are a spirit that lives in a body that possesses a soul. Sickness can start in any one part of our three-fold being; but often it ultimately affects all three areas. Medical science usually only focuses on the body and perchance the soul (mind, will and emotions) but as Christians, ministering to the spirit-man is vital when caring for our sick loved ones. A spiritual approach to caregiving transforms it into ministry. 3 John 1:2 implies that spiritual prosperity brings healing physically & emotionally. As a caregiver, God can use you to minister spiritually as well as physically and emotionally to your loved one. One of the definitions of ministering is to give service, care or aid; to attend to wants or necessities. When you use a spiritual approach to care for your sick loved ones, you are giving service, you are attending to their wants, needs and necessities. You are ministering.

EMOTIONALLY

Sick people are often in pain
Sick people are often grumpy
Sick people are often sharp-tongued
Sick people are often snappy
Sick people are often tearful
Sick people are often whinny
Sick people are often touchy
Sick people are often withdrawn
Sick people are often depressed
Sick people are often weak
Sick people are often downtrodden
Sick people are often scared or fearful
Sick people are often self-centered
Sick people are often slow to respond
Sick people often look or act mean
Sick people lack hope, are full of doubt & often feel like giving up.

These emotions can affect the caregiver and can transfer onto the caregiver's state of mind if allowed.

PRACTICALLY

Taking care of a sick loved one can be demanding, draining and depressing, especially if you have not been trained to do so. Most people who find themselves in this dilemma don't realize they are not in the situation alone. They don't realize there is help available.

  This booklet inspires to help you, support you, and equip you to give compassionate care (spirit, soul and body) to your loved one at home. This booklet inspires to provide helpful information and resources available to assist you as you perform the Ministry of Caregiving.

Care-giving 101

Sick loved ones can be hard to deal with. Sick loved ones may be forgetful, disoriented to place, time or person. They may be totally confused. In the final stages of illness, loved ones can become lethargic or non-responsive. Their joints may become contracted (unbendable or frozen). They may have open sores. They may be in a semi-comatose or a full comatose state. They may eventually reach a state where they are unable to be maintained at home. But most family members prefer to care for their loved ones at home as long as possible. The difficulty of caring for a chronically sick loved one at home can be lessened if one has the right attitude, proper resources, and the proper information on how to provide care without becoming bitter, angry or even sick as the caregiver. It is possible to care for your loved one as service unto Christ our Lord; but to minister to your loved one as unto the Lord, you must provide compassionate care.

What is compassionate care?

Compassion is a verb. It prompts an action. It prompts a response to bring improvement to a situation. Unlike sympathy, compassion is not looking at a situation and just feeling sorry for an individual. Compassion is actively getting involved in the individual's dilemma. Compassion is understanding. Compassion is treating that person as if you shared their pain or were capable of facing a similar dilemma. It involves treating another like you would like to be treated with kindness, dignity, respect and assistance. It was demonstrated by the Good Samaritan, who not only helped the wounded and injured traveler but took an active, positive role in the restoration and recovery of the traveler's health and wellness (Luke 10:25–37).

Compassion is treating others the way Jesus commissioned us, when He said "when I was sick, you comforted me…you gave me a glass of water (Matthew 25:35-36).

Compassion is following Jesus commission demonstrated by His words, "whatsoever ye do to the least of these…" (Matthew 25:40). True compassion will always eliminate resentment, despair, and abuse when providing care.

The Tasks of Care-giving

Caring for a loved one at home, involves the same skills used by a certified nursing assistant, home health aide or nurse. It involves bedbaths if your loved one is unable to be placed in a bathtub or shower. It involves providing proper hygiene, skincare, mouthcare, footcare (this is essential if your loved one is a diabetic) and may include wound care & dressings if the skin is not intact. Homecare requires bedmaking, feeding, meal preparation, proper nutrition, and transferring from the bed, wheelchair and/or toilet. It could require the use of a bedpan, catheter or urinal.

Agencies are usually available to give you some assistance; but as a home caregiver, many of these tasks will be done by the family member when the agency worker is not present or unavailable. Agencies that assist with caring for your loved one at home are vital resources. They provide care for your loved one, provide respite relief (times of rest for the caregiver), and can give training and instruction to the family member (Please see index for list of agencies that can assist you. Please see index for a Personal Care Task List)

Tools for the Task

The degree of sickness or condition of your loved one will determine what equipment and supplies are needed for their care. The most basic items include:

- Incontinence Briefs (i.e. Depends)
- Geriatric Skincare Products (i.e. Peri-wash)
- Blood Pressure Monitor
- Glucose Monitor for Diabetes (i.e. Accu-Chek)
- Bed Pads (Washable or Disposable)
- Waterproof Mattress Cover
- Wash Cloths or Wipes
- Bathtub Mat
- Weight Scale
- Elevated Toilet Seat
- Bed Rails
- Cane or Walker
- Recliner Chair or Lift Chair
- Thermometer

Other items that may be needed as need for care progresses may include:

- Wheelchair
- Hospital Bed
- Bedside Commode or Bedpan
- Shower Chair
- Grab Bars
- Hoyer-Lift
- Stair-Lifts

Another important tool that assists in good caregiving includes knowing the signs of the need for medical intervention. There will be times when you will need to call the doctor's office or emergency room for professional advice. These following signs require immediate attention and/or advice from a medical professional:

- Nosebleeds
- Blood Pressure Issues (lower than 70/50, greater than 180/100)
- Blood Sugar Issues (lower than 60, greater than 200)
- Excessive sweating
- Prolonged Fever (greater than 101.5)
- Low Body Temperature (lower than 96.)
- Excessive Weakness or Inability to Walk
- Sudden Confusion/Disorientation
- Slurred Speech
- Weakness on One Side of the Body
- Dizziness
- Blurred Vision
- Dark, Smelly Urine
- Bedsores/Open Wounds
- Excessive Diarrhea
- Rash
- Excessive Constipation (no bowel movement for more than 2-3 days)
- Dehydration (low fluid intake: resulting in dry lips. dry tongue or dry mouth, wrinkled & saggy skin, sudden confusion, weakness, decrease in skin elasticity, racing heartbeat or heartrate, sunken eyes, inability to produce tears, dizziness, feeling faint or light-headed…)

Other symptoms that require medical attention:

- Shallow breathing
- Difficulty breathing
- Lethargy (extreme sleepiness, hard to arouse)
- Prolonged extremity pain, spasms or cramps (frequent charley horse pain could actually be signs of a blood clot)
- Call 911 if loved one is not breathing or unconscious

Important Spiritual Tools

- Allowing the Holy Spirit to minister thru you and to you
- Prayer
- The Fruit of the Spirit (Galatians 5:22-23)
- The Royal Law (James 2:8)
- Positive Daily Confessions
- Biblical Decrees, Proclamations and Declarations
- Standing on God's Promises (purchase a Bible Promise Book)
- A Peaceful Atmosphere
- Worship Music
- Praise Music
- A Loving and Caring Attitude
- Ministering Angels (including those who come in the form of friends or family with CNA or Personal Care training or just someone with a willing heart to help in whatsoever manner they can)
- THE WORD OF GOD

Difficulties that may arise in the Ministry of Caregiving

Jesus said, in this life we may have trouble, be of good cheer for I have overcome the world. Test and trials can arise even as you go about the ministry of caregiving. Often times if unresolved or unspoken issues exist among the family members, these issues will surface during the care of your loved one.

- Issues of perceived unfairness in the sharing of the care duties.
- Anger and strife as a result of the stress sometimes associated with caregiving, especially as your loved one loses more and more of their independence, requiring difficult lifting & other backbreaking tasks.
- Backbiting and competition among the caregivers as the stress and strain weighs on
- Criticism from involved and uninvolved family members
- The possibility of loss of property and bank accounts if nursing home placement is required
- The list can go on and on

When Sibling or Relative Difficulties Arise

It is during this time that one called to the ministry of the caregiver must remember that their service is unto the Lord and unto their ill or sick loved one. It is a time of intense testing, but a test that can be overcome if the focus is placed back upon the Lord and the ministry to your loved one. You must remember to stay focused.   Do not allow others to inflict stress, strain and unreasonable demands upon you as you provide compassionate care to your loved one.

Sometimes the stress, the strain, and the difficulty comes as an indication that your loved one's situation may need to be re-assessed for professional intervention or help.

Taking care of yourself while in the ministry of care-giving

When caring for your loved one at home, it is especially important that you also take care of yourself.

Too many times, caregivers become sick themselves because they allow the ministry of caregiving to become a difficult task, allowing drain and strain to wear them down. Caregivers must get:

- Proper sleep
- drink plenty of water
- take vitamins or supplements
- eat 2 – 3 meals a day
- laugh
- Smile
- pray
- Worship
- Praise
- read the Word of God
- Interact with other believers who are outside the home for encouragement.

At least once every month attend a worship service at your local church. An alternative would be Christian TV if it is entirely impossible for you to find a substitute caregiver, family member or friend to relieve you. Daily Bible reading is a must for the ministry of caregiving as it provides strength and encouragement. Even reading for 10 – 20 minutes a day is beneficial. An alternative to reading is to listen to the Bible on Tape. This not only blesses you but your loved one as well. If times get really tough, take the time to fast and pray.

Always remember, in the ministry of caregiving it is important to take one day at a time. Each day brings a fresh start. Forget about the mistakes or failures of yesterday and start afresh each day. (Remember Lamentations 3:23 "His mercies are new every morning, Great is God's faithfulness).

What if my loved one is placed in the Hospital?

Should your loved one require hospitalization, it is important to visit during the doctor's rounds and be available to ask questions, as well as provide information. If this is not possible, you can usually find a pleasant nurse who will call the on-call doctor to address your concerns. In the hospital setting, you and the professional care staff are a team. Your input is important, as you are now in the role of advocate for your loved one. You are the administrator for your loved ones needs; so keep asking questions and making requests until you are satisfied. And speaking in love, make changes as often as you like. It is also important to ask questions about any treatments or dressing changes that may occur once your loved one returns home. Don't be afraid to ask 'why' your loved one needs a particular service, procedure, type of equipment, assessment, re-evaluation or change in medication. Be led by the Spirit of God. Ask about anything you do not understand. Be especially diligent to ask about:

- wound care & dressing change procedures
- Ostomy care and supplies
- Trach care and supplies
- Any other type of treatment you are unfamiliar with or uncomfortable about.

Question and inform the doctor should you feel ill prepared for your loved ones discharge from the hospital. Be adamant that you are properly instructed by the staff, so that you will be fully prepared and adequately trained to provide any and all pertinent care tasks needed by your loved one upon the return home. Also make sure you are properly trained to use any equipment sent home with your loved one.

What if my loved one is suffering from Alzheimer's/Dementia

Alzheimer's and/or Dementia care may be one of the most challenging type of caregiving. It is illness that affects the brain. It is now known that the brain actually shrinks when this disease attacks and gradually incapacitates its victims. There are also chemical changes that occur in addition to the physical shrinking.

There is hope. Much research in normal aging, early dementia, mid-stage dementia, late stage dementia and last stage dementia including Alzheimer's disease has occurred and the resources available are promising and vast. One of the best resources for this type of caregiving can be found at the website of Teepa Snow. (Visit www.teepasnow.com)

What if my loved one suffers from Parkinson's Disease?

Another challenging and gradually debilitating illness is Parkinson's. There has also been much research for this illness and many resources available. It's symptoms of shaking, stiffness, slowness and unsteadiness will make caregiving challenging and will require much patience especially for bathing, dressing and preventing falls. Resources are available thru National Parkinson Foundation (www.parkinson.org). Also visit www.pdf.org and www.apdaparkinson.com for further resources.

What if my loved one needs home health services or senior companion care services?

Often after release from the hospital, Home Health or Senior Companion Services may be required for your loved one to be discharged without 24 hour supervision at home. The Home Health Agency will visit for an assessment and often will ask you "what do you need?" Often first-time caregivers don't know what they need or what to expect. Even if you are told what you will need, frequently it is not until after you actually go through an experience that you fully understand why you need a particular service, procedure, type of equipment, re-assessment, evaluation or medication change. Keep asking questions and making all requests known until you feel comfortable. And make changes as often as you like. If necessary request a different Home Health Service, if you are not satisfied. You are the true administrator for your loved one's needs; and your loved one should receive the best care and attention possible. You are your loved one's best advocate because you know your loved one better than anyone. Don't be intimidated by a title, you have the Holy Spirit guiding you.

What if I have to place my loved one in Rehab or a nursing home?

There may come a time, when for the safety of yourself and your loved one, that you may have to place your loved one in a nursing facility or rehabilitation center. At times these placements may be temporary, until your loved one gains the wellness and the strength to return home. At other times, these placements may be a permanent solution to the best care for your loved one. The number one issue is the safety and well-being of your loved one. Placement in a facility will require you to research and investigate the reputation of the potential nursing or rehabilitation center. Just as God has guided you in the care of your loved one at home, God is able to guide you in finding a loving and caring nursing or rehabilitation facility.

Facilities types include private and family-run facilities, large corporate facilities, as well as, state and federally-run facilities. After choosing a facility, one way to ensure the best care for your loved one is to visit often. Share visiting assignments with family members and friends. If possible, have someone visit after breakfast and another person to visit during therapy sessions, and another after lunch, and another after dinner or before bedtime. When families visit on a regular and consistent basis, facilities seem to give better care to your loved one. This possibly is because the staff develops a relationship with the family because of the consistent presence of family and/or friends

What if my loved one is placed on Hospice or Palliative Care?

When one is not expected to live beyond six months, they are placed in Hospice Care; it provides comfort measures only. Hospice provides no prevention measures, no curative care, nor any emergency interventions; the sole focus is to keep your loved one out of pain and discomfort. Its goal is to provide a soothing atmosphere in which your loved one may gradually transition into eternal rest. Terms used in Hospice Care include DNR, which stands for do not resuscitate and NPO which stands for nothing by mouth. It is usually in the final days of life that NPO is implemented; as comfort measures in the early stages of Hospice allow for measured amounts of water and food for comfort, nourishment and skin integrity. Often the medication morphine is used in Hospice care to alleviate pain and discomfort; it also slows the heart & breathing. At times other medications are used to decrease agitation that sometimes occurs. As believers, we know that soothing worship music, comforting scriptures and gentle touch are a great comfort to loved ones at this stage of transition. Be led by the Holy Spirit as you minister to your loved one. Also be led by the Holy Spirit concerning what or how your Hospice Services are provided. You still remain in control regarding the care of your loved one and have a say in the determination of what is in your loved ones best interest. There are many Christian Hospice services, so carefully choose who will provide the services for your loved ones final days. (visit www.hrrv.org or call (800) 237-4629 for additional Hospice related information.)

Palliative Care

Palliative Care is for anyone with a serious illness. You can have Palliative Care Services at any age and any stage of a debilitating, painful illness; and you can have it along with curative treatment and care. It is not dependent on prognosis as in Hospice Care. (visit http://getpalliativecare.org for more information on Palliative Care.)

Should the Lord take your loved one to their heavenly home

- Know that you did your part with the help of the Lord
- know that you 'ministered' to your loved one in the giving of compassionate care
- Know that God is in control of times and seasons regarding your loved ones illness and eternal homegoing
- Know that gifts and callings are of the Lord, and it was God who called you to your season of the ministry of compassionate caregiving to His glory

It is also important to take time after the death of your loved one, to not only grieve the death, but to grieve the loss of your role as a caregiver. This phase of the caregiving ministry requires the same spiritual tools and helps that sustained you while you were caring for your loved one. You will need to continue to meditate on the Word of God. You will need to continue to sit in the presence of the Holy Spirit, as well as continue in prayer, Biblical confessions, decrees and declarations. You will need to continue to stand on God's Promises and continue to maintain a peaceful atmosphere thru praise and worship music.

The Reward

No one knows how long their assignment will be as a minister of caregiving. But one thing is known and that is you will be rewarded by God for your labor of love. You will find that as you are ministering to your sick loved one, God will be at work in you, teaching and guiding you into increased intimacy with Himself. The greatest reward for a Christian is to really know God. Intimacy produces that knowing. The ministry of caregiving has produced many good and faithful servants because of the intimacy that was developed as they relied upon God to minister to their loved one.

God has special regard for the poor, the downtrodden and the sick. And God has special regard for those called to care for the poor, the downtrodden, and the sick; especially when it involves beloved, sick family members. Care-giving is a commission. You have been called and chosen by God. Remember 'Care-giving' is a ministry and God is able to supply you with the emotional, spiritual, and practical skills needed to perform this task in love.

Index I

Personal Care

The following areas must be incorporated into your loved ones care schedule to promote quality and restorative care. Many use a schedule and/or calendar of events to ensure good healthcare for their loved one:

- Bathtub or Shower (once or twice weekly)
- Bedbath or Bedside-bath (daily)
- Mouthcare (daily)
- Shampoo (weekly)
- Skincare (daily includes cleaning and lotioning of the skin)
- Haircare (daily combing and brushing)
- Nailcare (as needed: please note diabetes require professional podiatrist treatment)
- Dressings (must be changed regularly as prescribed by MD & must always be clean, pus-free and discharge-free to prevent infection)
- Range of motion/movement of joints (daily to prevent contractures or frozen joints)
- Ambulation as much as possible for those able to walk (encouraged to maintain mobility)
- Position changes (side to back to opposite side rotation for bedridden loved ones every 2-3 hours, this prevents bedsores)
- Toileting/Diapering (check every 2 – 3 hours to maintain bladder control and skin integrity)
- Feeding and hydration (regular meals and fluids prevents malnutrition & dehydration)

- Communication (clock, calendar, newspaper, crossword puzzles, current events... to promote orientation of person, place, time, day, month & year, etc. and mental stimulation)
- Males require regular shaving and beard trimming

Use self-care assistive devices to promote as much independence as possible according to your loved ones capability. These include: long handled shoe horns, grabbers, raised spoons/forks, other adaptive equipment, etc.

Index II

Resources for the Ministry of Caregiving
There are agencies who provide many of the tasks and
services previously listed, please make use of all available
resources. There is help available in the form of Nursing
support, CNA assistance, Home Health aides, Companion
Care aides, caregiver training for family members, social
service support, emotional support and respite care. In the
Ministry of Caregiving, always remember your greatest help
is the Lord!

National Assistance
United States Administration on Aging - Official Site

www.aoa.gov

(also visit) Benefits.gov - Caregiver Programs and Services

AARP
www.aarp.com/caregiver

State Assistance

Each State has a Department of Aging. Please contact your state's department for resources and services in your state. Please access thru your state's official website.
Also most states have an Association of Area Agencies on Aging. They provide information about resources and service providers, assessments, referrals, case managers, links to services & monitors consumer satisfaction. To be connected with your local Area Agency on Aging, just call 800-986-3505.

Local Assistance

Caregiver Homes (www.caregiverhomes.org)
This organization provides what is known as structured family caregiving. It provides coaching, support & financial assistance to the family caregiver. It currently is available in Indiana, Ohio, Massachusetts, Connecticut and Louisiana with other states in the developing stages.

Senior Helpers (www.seniorhelpers.com)
This organization specializes in Alzheimer's/Dementia and Parkinson's care. It also provides companion and/or personal care in the home, assisted living facility, etc. Local offices are available in most cities. Call 800-760-6389 for in-home or facility assistance.

Master's Touch Home Care, LLC (317-672-7634)
(www.dmoore@masterstouchhc.com)
A local company of registered nurses, licensed practical nurses, certified nursing assistants, home health aides and social workers to assure your loved ones gets compassionate and loving care.

Christian Resources & Agencies

www.christiancaregiversupport.com
This organization provides devotional readings, current articles from across the web, as well as information on how to start a Christian Caregiver Support Group. It is home to "The Christian Caregiver Blog" and provides many other resources for the Christian caregiver.

www.restministries.org/life/caregiver.htm
This organization provides information for various online Caregiver Support Ministries and organizations. It provides access to resources, conferences, tools & articles to assist caregivers.

Index III

Scripture Helps for the Caregiver

1.   …Isaiah 42:3 (gentleness & sensitivity)
2.   …Matthew 19:19 (honor & love)
3.   …Romans 13:10 (love & care)
4.   …Galatians 6:2 (compassion)
5.   …1 Timothy 1:5 (charity)
6.   …Leviticus 19:18 (mercy)
7.   …Matthew 7:12 (mercy)
8.   …Psalm 23 (trust)
9.   …Psalm 22:19 (patience)
10.   …Isaiah 46:4 (grace)
11.   …Isaiah 50:4 (comfort)
12.   …Proverbs 12:25 (encouragement)
13.   …Isaiah 40:29 (strength)
14.   …Isaiah 58:8 (healing)
15.   …Jeremiah 17:14 (healing)
16.   …Malachi 4:2 (healing)
17.   …2 Chronicles 20:15, 17 (divine help)
18.   …Psalm 20:7 (trust)
19.   …Psalm 118:8 (trust)
20.   …Zechariah 4:6 (strength)
21.   …Isaiah 41:10 (courage)
22.   …Proverb 12:25 (encouragement)
23.   …Romans 15:5 (encouragement)
24.   …1Peter 3:8 (compassion)
25.   …2 Corinthians 1:3-4 (comfort)
26.   …Isaiah 61:1-2 (comfort)
27.   …Isaiah 42:7 (comfort)
28.   …Psalm 34:18 (comfort)
29.   …Psalm 147:3 (healing)

30.   ...Psalm 107:19-21 (healing)
31.   ...Psalm 30:2 (redemption)
32.   ...Hebrews 4:16 (mercy & grace)
33.   ...Psalm 28:8 (strength)
34.   ...Habakkuk 3:19 (strength)
35.   ...Psalm 28:7, 8 (strength)
36.   ...1 Chronicles 16:11 (strength)
37.   ...Psalm 67:1 (mercy)
38.   ...3 John 1:2 (prosperity)
39.   ...Jeremiah 33:6 (healing)
40.   ...Proverbs 16:24 (health)

Much comfort can be found in the scriptures especially the Psalms. Allow the Holy Spirit to speak to you and lead you in the comfort that only comes from God's Word. Seek out the healing scriptures of the Bible for you and your loved one.

You can believe for your Loved Ones healing

Healing Scriptures: Decree these scriptures over your loved one as "God's Medicine".

Jeremiah 30:17 "For I will restore health to you, and I will heal your wounds, says the Lord…

Psalm 103:3 "He forgives all your sin; He heals all your diseases"

Jeremiah 33:6 "Yet I will certainly bring health and healing to it and will indeed heal them. I will let them experience the abundance of peace and truth."

Psalm 107:20 "He sent His word and healed them; He rescued them from the Pit."

Deuteronomy 7:15a "The Lord will remove all sickness from you…"

Jeremiah 17:14 "Heal me, Lord, and I will be healed; save me, and I will be saved, for You are my praise"

Isaiah 53:5 "But He was pierced because of our transgressions, crushed because of our iniquities; punishment for our peace was on Him, and we are healed by His wounds."

Psalm 41:2-3 "The Lord will keep him and preserve him; he will be blessed in the land. You will not give him over to the desire of his enemies. The Lord will sustain him on his sickbed; You will heal him on the bed where he lies. "

Psalm 34:19 "Many adversities (sickness, infirmity, disease...) come to the one who is righteous, but the Lord delivers him from them all.

Exodus 15:26 "He said, "If you will carefully obey the Lord your God, do what is right in His eyes, pay attention to His commands, and keep all His statutes, I will not inflict any illnesses on you that I inflicted on the Egyptians. For I am Yahweh who heals you."

Exodus 23:25 "Worship the Lord your God, and He[a] will bless your bread and your water. I will remove illnesses from you."

Psalm 147:3 "He heals the brokenhearted and binds up their wounds. "

Proverbs 4:20-22 "My son, pay attention to my words; listen closely to my sayings. Don't lose sight of them; keep them within your heart. For they are life to those who find them, and health to one's whole body."

1 Peter 2:24 "He Himself bore our sins in His body on the tree, so that, having died to sins, we might live for righteousness; you have been healed by His wounds "

Psalm 30:2 Lord my God, I cried to You for help, and You healed me. "

Matthew 8:17 "so that what was spoken through the prophet Isaiah might be fulfilled: He Himself took our weaknesses and carried our diseases.

Proverbs 9:11 "For by Wisdom your days will be many, and years will be added to your life. "
Psalm 91:10 "no harm will come to you; no plague will come near your tent "

3 John 2 "Dear friend, I pray that you may prosper in every way and be in good health physically just as you are spiritually.

(God's Medicine compiled by Apostle Kevin Bailey, Touch of the Master Healing Ministries INTL)

Prayers Helps for the Ministry of Caregiving

Heavenly Father, in the Name of our Lord and Savior Jesus Christ and by the power of the Holy Spirit, I make my requests and petitions known to you today. I thank you for your promises and I stand on Your Word. I am grateful that Your Word does not return void, but it accomplishes what you please and prospers in the thing for which you have sent it. I thank You that You sent Your Word and it provides healing, comfort, peace, strength, wisdom, knowledge, understanding and supernatural ability to me today. I thank you that I can do all things thru Christ who strengthens me. I thank you for the strength to care for my love one this day. I thank you for strengthening my loved one today. I thank you for comforting my loved one today. I thank you for giving myself and my loved one peace today. I thank you for giving me wisdom to perform the tasks needed this day to care for my loved one. I thank you for divine knowledge and the insight to meet the needs of my loved one today. Thank You for giving me an understanding, patient, kind and compassionate heart today. Thank You for divine ability today and for angelic assistance in providing empathic care for my loved one. Lord, I thank you that Your Word is a lamp unto my feet and a light unto my path. Thank You for leading me and guiding in the paths of righteousness, thank You for restoring my soul and the soul of my loved one. Thank You for removing all fear from myself and my loved one. You promised never to leave me nor forsake me. You promised to be with me. So I stand on your promises today. And I look to you for guidance in all that I must accomplish today.

Heavenly Father, In the Name of my Lord and Savior Jesus Christ and by the power of the Holy Spirit, I decree and declare Your Word. You said "Whatever I shall BIND on earth, shall be BOUND in heaven and whatsoever I LOOSE on earth, shall be LOOSED in Heaven...so today I bind sickness and disease in Jesus Name. I bind infirmity and pain in Jesus Name. I bind oppression in Jesus Name. I bind all spirits of death and destruction in Jesus Name. I rebuke sickness and command it to go in the Name of Jesus Christ. I speak life and loose the healing virtue of Jesus Christ into the systems of my loved one. I speak life unto the cardiovascular system, respiratory system, endocrine system, circulatory system, digestive system, nervous system, skeletal system and all organs; I do this by faith and in the power and authority in Jesus Name. Amen

Heavenly Father, In the Name of Jesus and by the power of the Holy Ghost, I decree and declare I can do all things thru Christ who strengthens me. I stand on your promises that You will never leave me nor forsake me. I stand on your promise for perfect peace as I keep my mind on You. Heavenly Father, release ministering angels into this home today as I go about the tasks of caring for my loved one. Give me the strength I need to give loving care. Remind me that in all I do today I do as unto You. I thank You for Your grace, Your mercy, Your comfort, Your strength, Your endurance and Your ability. Allow my loved one to feel Your love through my ministry of caregiving. Let me represent You as I perform each task. I bind up murmuring, complaining, criticism, apathy, fear and all hindrances that would attempt to interfere with my tasks today. Thank You Lord for supernatural ability and an anointing to complete every task with love and compassion. Amen

Additional Helps

Visit www.christianword.org for a free little red prayer book (you may download or request paperback for a small donation).

Also a personal prayer journal is a wonderful way to submit your prayers to God as you minister in caregiving.

Also prayer lines are available to uplift you in prayer:

Joan Hunter Prayer Line: 281-789-7500
http://joanhunter.org

700 Club Prayer Center: 800-700-7000
https://www1.cbn.com

Made in the USA
Middletown, DE
20 September 2020

19158800R00022